Comprehensive Anti Inflammatory Recipe Collection

Fit and Healthy Side Dishes Recipes to Boost your Metabolism

Mya Castillo

Table of Contents

Garden Vegetable Mash

Prep Time:
15 minutes
Serve: 3

Ingredients:

- 1 ½ tablespoons butter
- 4 tablespoons cream cheese
- ½ pound cauliflower florets
- ½ pound broccoli florets
- 1/2 teaspoon garlic powder

Directions:

1.Parboil the broccoli and cauliflower for about 10 minutes until they have softened. Mash them with a potato masher.

2.Add in garlic powder, cream cheese, and butter; mix to combine well. Season with salt and black pepper to taste.

Nutrition: 162 Calories; 12.8g Fat; 7.2g Carbs; 4.7g Protein; 3.5g Fiber

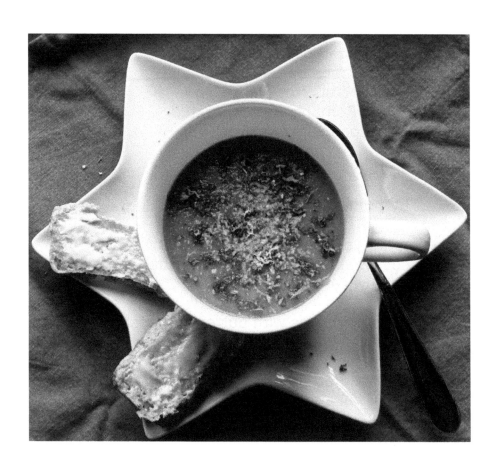

Spicy and Cheesy Roasted Artichokes

Prep Time:
1 hour 10 minutes
Serve: 2

Ingredients:

- 2 small-sized globe artichokes, cut off the stalks
- 2 tablespoons butter, melted
- 2 tablespoons fresh lime juice
- 1/2 cup Romano cheese, grated
- 2 tablespoons mayonnaise

Directions:

1.Start by preheating your oven to 420 degrees F.

2.To prepare your artichokes, discard the tough outer layers; cut off about 3/4 inches from the top. Slice them in half lengthwise.

3.Toss your artichokes with butter and fresh lime juice; season with the salt and pepper to taste.

4.Top with the grated Romano cheese; wrap your artichokes in foil and roast them in the preheated oven for about 1 hour.

Nutrition: 368 Calories; 33g Fat; 7.2g Carbs; 10.6g Protein; 3.8g Fiber

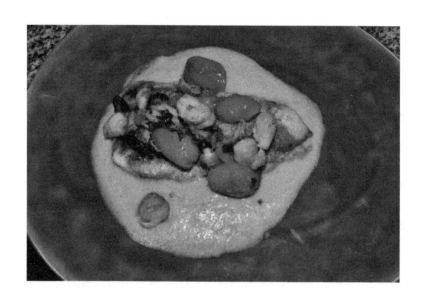

Cheesy Stuffed Peppers with Cauliflower Rice

Prep Time:
45 minutes
Serve: 6

Ingredients:

- 6 medium-sized bell peppers, deveined and cleaned
- 1 cup cauliflower rice
- 1/2 cup tomato sauce with garlic and onion
- 1 pound ground turkey
- 1/2 cup Cheddar cheese, shredded

Directions:

1.Heat 2 tablespoons of olive oil in a frying pan over medium-high heat. Then, cook ground turkey until nicely browned or about 5 minutes.

2.Add in cauliflower rice and season with salt and black p epper. Continue to cook for 3 to 4 minutes more.

3.Add in tomato sauce. Stuff the peppers with this filling and cover with a piece of aluminum foil.

4.Bake in the preheated oven at 390 degrees F for 17 to 20 minutes. Remove the foil, top with cheese, and bake for a further 10 to 13 minutes. Bon appétit!

Nutrition: 244 Calories; 12.9g Fat; 3.2g Carbs; 1g Fiber; 16.5g Protein;

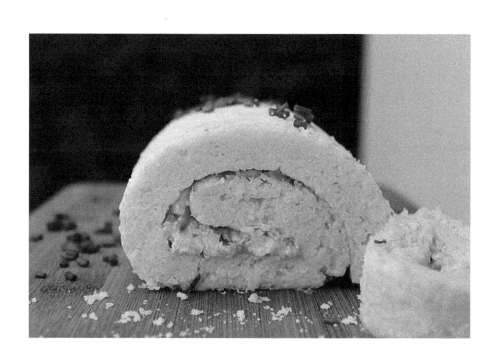

Broccoli and Bacon Soup

Prep Time:
20 minutes
Serve: 4

Ingredients:

- 1 head broccoli, broken into small florets
- 1 carrot, chopped
- 1 celery, chopped
- 1/2 cup full-fat yogurt
- 2 slices bacon, chopped

Directions:

1.Fry the bacon in a soup pot over a moderate flame; reserve.

2.Then, cook the carrots, celery and broccoli in the bacon fat. Season with salt and pepper to taste.

3.Pour in 4 cups of water or vegetable stock, bringing to a boil. Turn the temperature to a simmer and continue to cook, partially covered, for 10 to 15 minutes longer.

4.Add in yogurt and remove from heat. Puree your soup with an immersion blender until your desired consistency is reached.

5.Garnish with the reserved bacon and serve.

Nutrition: 95 Calories; 7.6g Fat; 4.1g Carbs; 3g Protein; 1g Fiber

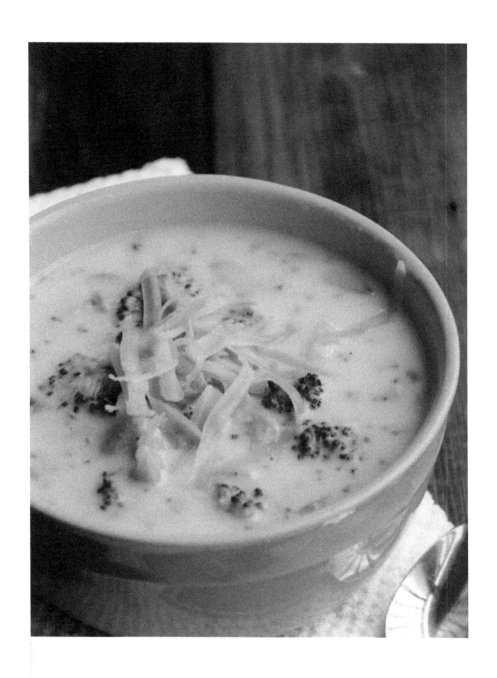

Aromatic Kale with Garlic

Prep Time:
20 minutes
Serve: 3

Ingredients:

- 1/2 tablespoon olive oil
- 1/2 cup cottage cheese, creamed
- 1/2 teaspoon sea salt
- 1 teaspoon fresh garlic, chopped
- 9 ounces kale, torn into pieces

Directions:

1.Heat the olive oil in a pot over medium-high flame. Once hot, fry the garlic until just tender and fragrant or about 30 seconds.

2.Add in kale and continue to cook for 8 to 10 minutes until all liquid evaporates.

3.Add in cottage cheese and sea salt, remove from heat, and stir until everything is combined. Bon appétit!

Nutrition: 93 Calories; 4.4g Fat; 6.1g Carbs; 7.1g Protein; 2.7g Fiber

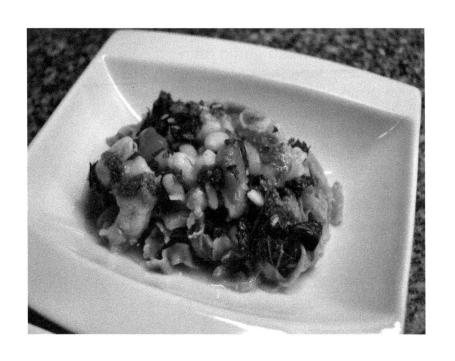

Spanish-Style Keto Slaw

Prep Time:
10 minutes
Serve: 4

Ingredients:

- 1 teaspoon fresh garlic, minced
- 4 tablespoons tahini (sesame paste
- ½ pound Napa cabbage, shredded
- 2 cups arugula, torn into pieces
- 1 Spanish onion, thinly sliced into rings

Directions:

1.Make a dressing by whisking the garlic and tahini; add in 2 teaspoons of balsamic vinegar along with salt and black pepper.

2.In a salad bowl, combine Napa cabbage, arugula, and Spanish onion. Toss the salad with dressing.

3.Garnish with sesame seeds if desired and serve.

Nutrition: 122 Calories; 9.1g Fat; 5.9g Carbs; 4.5g Protein; 3g Fiber

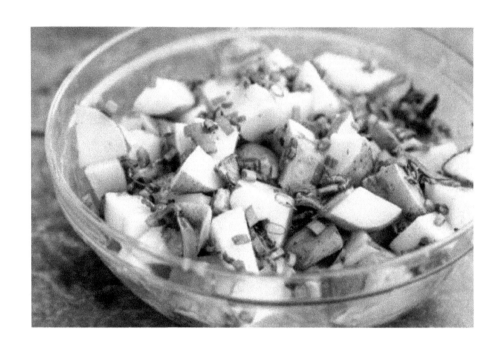

Cheesy Breakfast Broccoli Casserole

Prep Time:
40 minutes
Serve: 4

Ingredients:

- 1 (1/2-poundhead broccoli, broken into florets
- 1 cup cooked ham, chopped
- 1/2 cup Greek-style yogurt
- 1 cup Mexican cheese, shredded
- 1/2 teaspoon butter, melted

Directions:

1.Begin by preheating an oven to 350 degrees F. Now, butter the bottom and sides of a casserole dish with melted butter.

2.Cook broccoli for 6 to 7 minutes until it is "mashable". Mash the broccoli with a potato masher.

3.Now, stir in Greek-style yogurt, Mexican cheese, and cooked ham. Season with Mexican spice blend, if desired.

4.Press the cheese/broccoli mixture in the buttered casserole dish. Bake in the preheated oven for 20 to 23 minutes.

Nutrition: 188 Calories; 11.3g Fat; 5.7g Carbs; 14.9g Protein; 1.1g Fiber

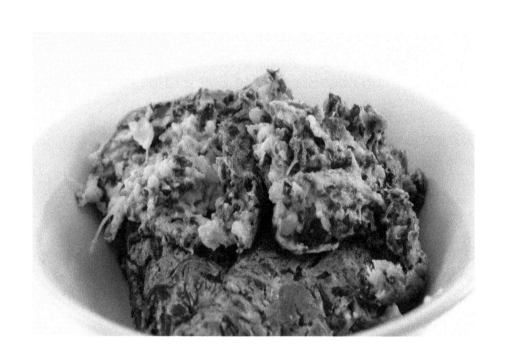

Cauli Mac and Cheese

Prep Time:
15 Minutes
Cook Time:
15 Minutes
Serve: 6

Ingredients:

- 1 head cauliflower, blanched and cut into florets
- ½ cup nutritional yeast
- 1 cup heavy cream
- 5 tablespoons butter, melted
- 1 ½ cup cheddar cheese Salt and pepper to taste
- ½ cup water or milk

Directions:

1.In a heat-proof dish, place the cauliflower florets. Set aside. In a mixing bowl, combine the rest of the ingredients. Pour over the cauliflower florets.

2.Bake in a 3500F preheated oven for 15 minutes. Place in containers and put the proper label. Store in the fridge and consume before 3 days. Microwave or bake in the oven first before eating.

Nutrition: Calories: 329; Fat: 30.3g; Carbs: 10.1g; Protein: 12.1g

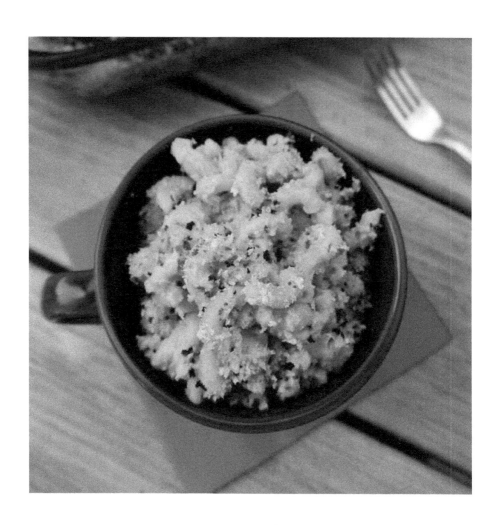

Baked Vegetable Side

Prep Time:
15 Minutes
Cook Time:
15 Minutes
Serve: 4

Ingredients:

- 2 large zucchinis, sliced
- 2 bell peppers, sliced
- ½ cup peeled garlic cloves, sliced A dash of oregano
- 4 tablespoons olive oil Salt and pepper to taste

Directions:

1.Place all ingredients in a mixing bowl. Stir to coat everything. Place in a baking sheet.

2.Bake in a 3500F preheated oven for 15 minutes.

Nutrition: Calories: 191; Fat: 23.0g; Carbs: 12.0g; Protein: 3.0g

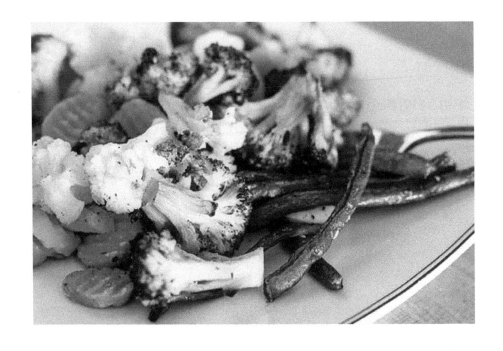

Shrimp Fra Diavolo

Prep Time:
15 Minutes
Cook Time:
5 Minutes
Serve: 3

Ingredients:

- 3 tablespoons butter
- 1 onion, diced
- 5 cloves of garlic, minced
- 1 teaspoon red pepper flakes
- ¼ pound shrimps, shelled
- 2 tablespoons olive oil Salt and pepper to taste

Directions:

1.Heat the butter and the olive oil in a skillet and sauté the onion and garlic until fragrant.

2.Stir in the red pepper flakes and shrimps. Season with salt and pepper to taste.

3.Stir for 3 minutes.

Nutrition: Calories: 145; Fat: 32.1g; Carbs: 4.5g; Protein: 21.0g

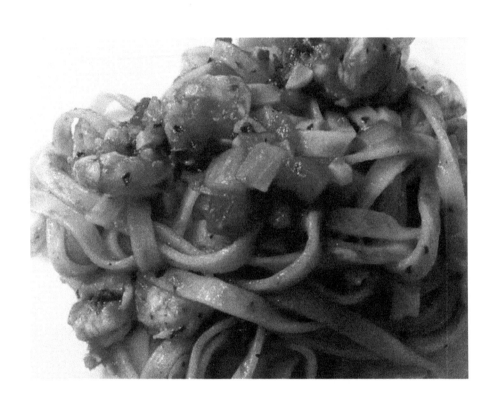

Zucchini and Cheese Gratin

Prep Time:
15 Minutes
Cook Time:
15 Minutes
Serve: 8

Ingredients:

- 5 tablespoons butter
- 1 onion, sliced
- ½ cup heavy cream
- 4 cups raw zucchini, sliced
- 1 ½ cups shredded pepper Jack cheese Salt and pepper to taste

Directions:

1.Place all ingredients in a mixing bowl and give a good stir to incorporate everything.

2.Pour the mixture in a heat-proof baking dish.

3.Place in a 3500F preheated oven and bake for 15 minutes.

Nutrition: Calories: 280; Fat: 20.0g; Carbs: 5.0g; Protein: 8.0g

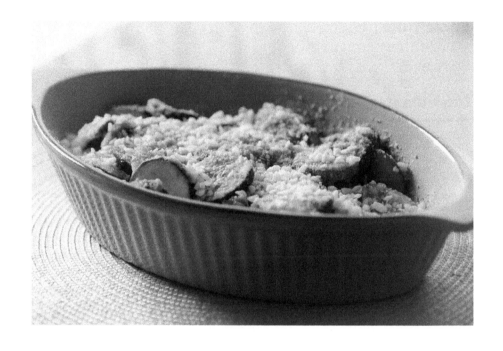

Soy Garlic Mushrooms

Prep Time:
20 Minutes
Cook Time:
10 Minutes
Serve: 8

Ingredients:

- 2 pounds mushrooms, sliced
- 3 tablespoons olive oil
- 2 cloves of garlic, minced
- ¼ncup coconut aminos Salt and pepper to taste

Directions:

1.Place all ingredients in a dish and mix until well-combined. Allow to marinate for 2 hours in the fridge.

2.In a large saucepan on medium fire, add mushrooms and sauté for 8 minutes.

3.Season with pepper and salt to taste.

Nutrition: Calories: 383; Fat: 10.9g; Carbs: 86.0g; Protein: 6.2g

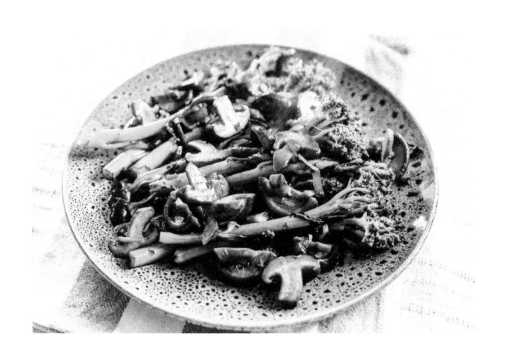

Old Bay Chicken Wings

Prep Time:
5 Minutes
Cook Time:
30 Minutes
Serve: 4

Ingredients:

- 3 pounds chicken wings
- ¾ cup almond flour
- 1 tablespoon old bay spices
- 1 teaspoon lemon juice, freshly squeezed
- ½ cup butter
- Salt and pepper to taste

Directions:

1.Preheat oven to 400oF.

2.In a mixing bowl, combine all ingredients except for the butter.

3.Place in an even layer in a baking sheet.

4.Bake for 30 minutes. Halfway through the cooking time, shake the fryer basket for even cooking.

5.Once cooked, drizzle with melted butter.

Nutrition: Calories: 640; Fat: 59.2g; Carbs: 1.6g; Protein: 52.5g

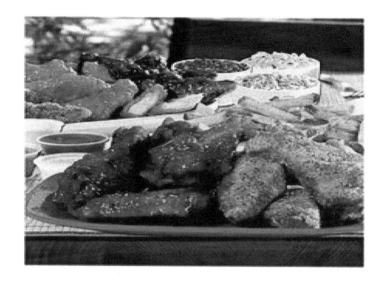

Tofu Stuffed Peppers

Prep Time:
5 Minutes
Cook Time:
10 Minutes
Serve: 8

Ingredients:

- 1 package firm tofu, crumbled
- 1 onion, finely chopped
- ½ teaspoon turmeric powder
- 1 teaspoon coriander powder
- 8 banana peppers, top end sliced and seeded Salt and pepper to taste
- 3 tablespoons oil

Directions:

1.Preheat oven to 400oF.

2.In a mixing bowl, combine the tofu, onion, coconut oil, turmeric powder, red chili powder, coriander power, and salt. Mix until well-combined.

3.Scoop the tofu mixture into the hollows of the banana peppers.

4.Place the stuffed peppers in one layer in a lightly greased baking sheet.

5.Cook for 10 minutes.

Nutrition: Calories: 67; Fat: 5.6g; Carbs: 4.1g; Protein: 1.2g

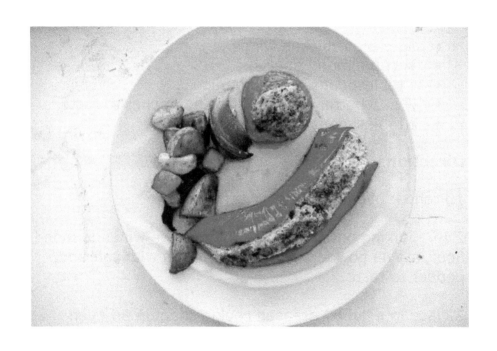

Air Fryer Garlic Chicken Wings

Prep Time:
5 Minutes
Cook Time:
25 Minutes
Serve: 4

Ingredients:

- 16 pieces chicken wings
- ¾ cup almond flour
- 4 tablespoons minced garlic
- ¼ cup butter, melted Salt and pepper to taste
- 2 tablespoons stevia powder

Directions:

1.Preheat oven to 400oF.

2.In a mixing bowl, combine the chicken wings, almond flour, stevia powder, and garlic Season with salt and pepper to taste.

3.Place in a lightly greased cookie sheet in an even layer and cook for 25 minutes.

4.Halfway through the cooking time, turnover chicken.

5.Once cooked, place in a bowl and drizzle with melted butter. Toss to coat.

Nutrition: Calories: 365; Fat: 26.9g; Carbs: 7.8g; Protein: 23.7g

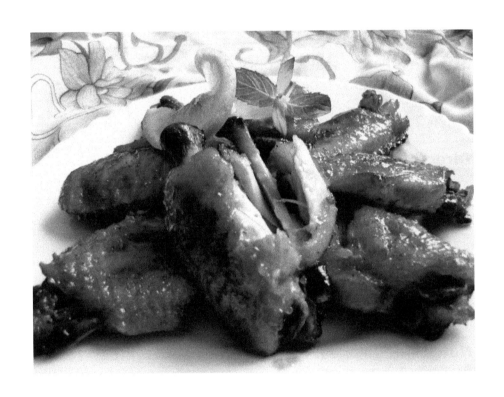

Sautéed Brussels Sprouts

Prep Time:
5 Minutes
Cook Time:
8 Minutes
Serve: 4

Ingredients:

- 2 cups Brussels sprouts, halved
- 1 tablespoon balsamic vinegar
- Salt and pepper to taste
- 2 tablespoons olive oil

Directions:

1.Place a saucepan on medium high fire and heat oil for a minute.

2.Add all ingredients and sauté for 7 minutes.

3.Season with pepper and salt.

Nutrition: Calories: 82; Fat: 6.8g; Carbs: 4.6g; Protein: 1.5g

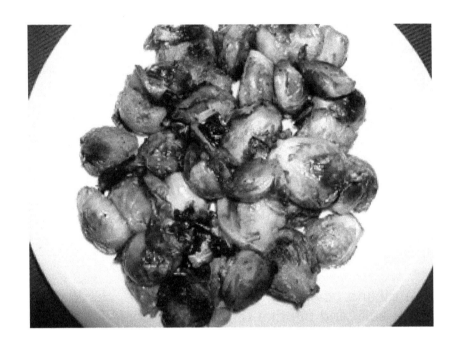

Bacon Jalapeno Poppers

Prep Time:
15 Minutes
Cook Time:
10 Minutes
Serve: 8

Ingredients:

- 4-ounce cream cheese
- ¼ cup cheddar cheese, shredded
- 1 teaspoon paprika
- 16 fresh jalapenos, sliced lengthwise and seeded
- 16 strips of uncured bacon, cut into half Salt and pepper to taste

Directions:

1.Preheat oven to 400oF.

2.In a mixing bowl, mix the cream cheese, cheddar cheese, salt, and paprika until well-combined.

3.Scoop half a teaspoon onto each half of jalapeno peppers.

4.Use a thin strip of bacon and wrap it around the cheese-filled jalapeno half.

5.Place in a single layer in a lightly greased baking sheet and roast for 10 minutes.

Nutrition: Calories: 225; Fat: 18.9g; Carbs: 3.2g; Protein: 10.6g

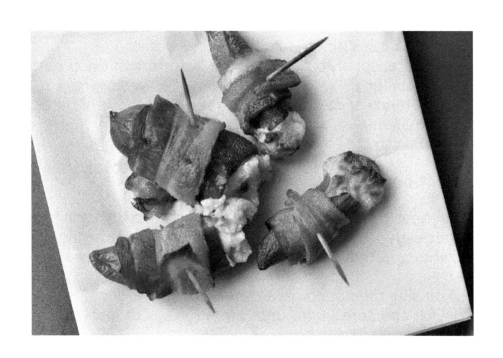

Basil Keto Crackers

Prep Time:
30 Minutes
Cook Time:
15 Minutes
Serve: 6

Ingredients:

- 1 ¼ cups almond flour
- ½ teaspoon baking powder ¼ teaspoon dried basil powder
- A pinch of cayenne pepper powder 1 clove of garlic, minced
- Salt and pepper to taste 3 tablespoons oil

Directions:

1.Preheat oven to 350oF and lightly grease a cookie sheet with cooking spray. Mix everything in a mixing bowl to create a dough.

2.Transfer the dough on a clean and flat working surface and spread out until 2mm thick. Cut into squares.

3.Place gently in an even layer on prepped cookie sheet. Cook for 10 minutes.

4.Cook in batches.

Nutrition: Calories: 205; Fat: 19.3g; Carbs: 2.9g; Protein: 5.3g

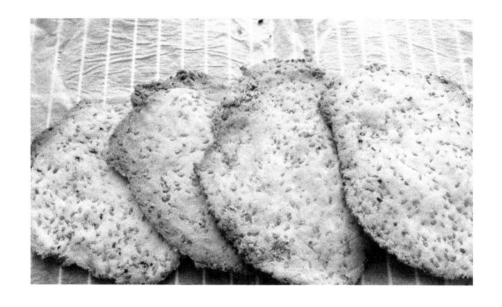

Crispy Keto Pork Bites

Prep Time:
20 Minutes
Cook Time:
30 Minutes
Serve: 3

- ½ pork belly, sliced to thin strips
- 1 tablespoon butter
- 1 onion, diced
- 4 tablespoons coconut cream Salt and pepper to taste

Directions:

1.Place all ingredients in a mixing bowl and allow to marinate in the fridge for 2 hours.

2.When 2 hours is nearly up, preheat oven to 400oF and lightly grease a cookie sheet with cooking spray.

3.Place the pork strips in an even layer on the cookie sheet. Roast for 30 minutes and turnover halfway through cooking.

Nutrition: Calories: 448; Fat: 40.6g; Carbs: 1.9g; Protein: 19.1g

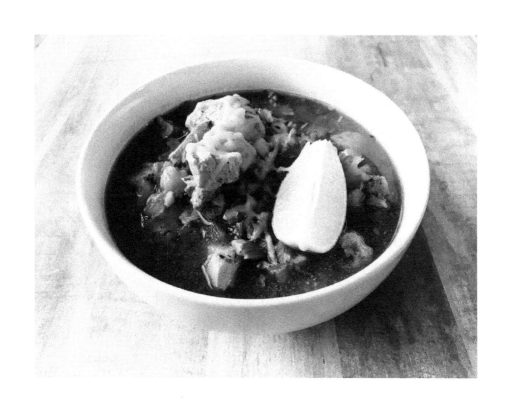

Fat Burger Bombs

Prep Time:
30 Minutes
Cook Time:
20 Minutes
Serve: 6

Ingredients:

- 12 slices uncured bacon, chopped
- 1 cup almond flour
- 2 eggs, beaten
- ½ pound ground beef Salt and pepper to taste
- 3 tablespoons olive oil

Directions:

1.In a mixing bowl, combine all ingredients except for the olive oil.

2.Use your hands to form small balls with the mixture. Place in a baking sheet and allow to set in the fridge for at least 2 hours.

3.Once 2 hours is nearly up, preheat oven to 400oF.

4.Place meatballs in a single layer in a baking sheet and brush the meat balls with olive oil on all sides.

5.Cook for 20 minutes.

Nutrition: Calories: 448; Fat: 40.6g; Carbs: 1.9g; Protein: 19.1g

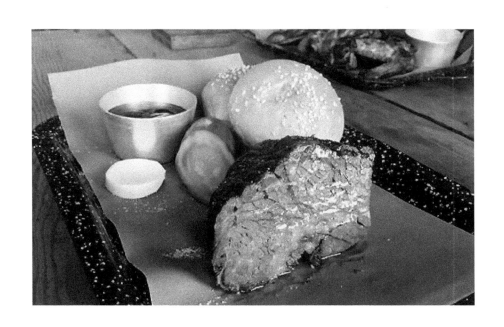

Onion Cheese Muffins

Prep Time:
20 Minutes
Cook Time:
20 Minutes
Serve: 6

Ingredients:

- ¼ cup Colby jack cheese, shredded
- ¼ cup shallots, minced
- 1 cup almond flour
- 1 egg
- 3 tbsp sour cream
- ½ tsp salt
- 3 tbsp melted butter or oil

Directions:

1.Line 6 muffin tins with 6 muffin liners. Set aside and preheat oven to 350oF.

2.In a bowl, stir the dry and wet ingredients alternately. Mix well using a spatula until the consistency of the mixture becomes even.

3.Scoop a spoonful of the batter to the prepared muffin tins.
Bake for 20 minutes in oven until golden brown.

Nutrition: Calories: 193; Fat: 17.4g; Carbs: 4.6g; Protein: 6.3g

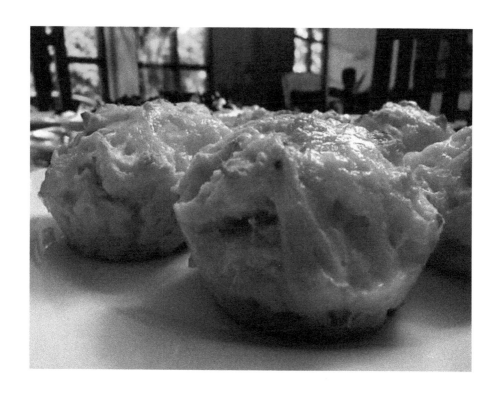

Bacon-Flavored Kale Chips

Prep Time:
20 Minutes
Cook Time:
25 Minutes
Serve: 6

Ingredients:

- 2 tbsp butter
- ¼ cup bacon grease
- 1-lb kale, around 1 bunch
- 1 to 2 tsp salt

Directions:

1.Remove the rib from kale leaves and tear into 2-inch pieces.

2.Clean the kale leaves thoroughly and dry them inside a salad spinner.

3.In a skillet, add the butter to the bacon grease and warm the two fats under low heat. Add salt and stir constantly.

4.Set aside and let it cool.

5.Put the dried kale in a Ziploc back and add the cool liquid bacon grease and butter mixture.

6.Seal the Ziploc back and gently shake the kale leaves with the butter mixture. The leaves should have this shiny consistency which means that they are coated evenly with the fat.

7.Pour the kale leaves on a cookie sheet and sprinkle more salt if necessary.

8.Bake for 25 minutes inside a preheated 350-degree oven or until the leaves start to turn brown as well as crispy.

Nutrition: Calories: 148; Fat: 13.1g; Carbs: 6.6g; Protein: 3.3g

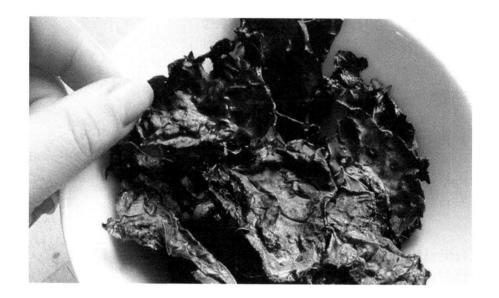

Keto-Approved Trail Mix

Prep Time:
10 Minutes
Cook Time:
3 Minutes
Serve: 8

Ingredients:

- ½ cup salted pumpkin seeds
- ½ cup slivered almonds
- ¾ cup roasted pecan halves
- ¾ cup unsweetened cranberries
- 1 cup toasted coconut flakes None

Directions:

1.In a skillet, place almonds and pecans. Heat for 2-3 minutes and let cool. Once cooled, in a large re-sealable plastic bag, combine all ingredients. Seal and shake vigorously to mix.

Nutrition: Calories: 184; Fat: 14.4g; Carbs: 13.0g; Protein: 4.4g

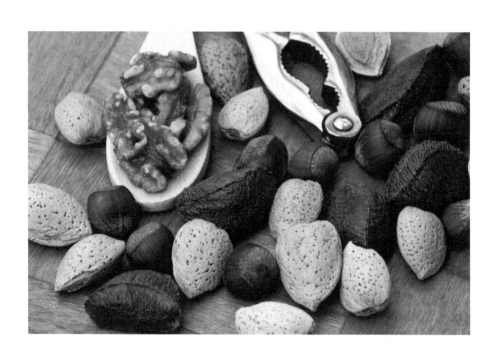

Reese Cups

Prep Time:
15 Minutes
Cook Time:
1 Min
Serve: 12

Ingredients:

- ½ cup unsweetened shredded coconut
- 1 cup almond butter
- 1 cup dark chocolate chips
- 1 tablespoon Stevia
- 1 tablespoon coconut oil

Directions:

1.Line 12 muffin tins with 12 muffin liners.

2.Place the almond butter, honey and oil in a glass bowl and microwave for 30 seconds or until melted. Divide the mixture into 12 muffin tins. Let it cool for 30 minutes in the fridge.

3.Add the shredded coconuts and mix until evenly distributed.

4.Pour the remaining melted chocolate on top of the coconuts. Freeze for an hour.

5.Carefully remove the chocolates from the muffin tins to create perfect Reese cups.

Nutrition: Calories: 214; Fat: 17.1g; Carbs: 13.7g; Protein: 5.0g

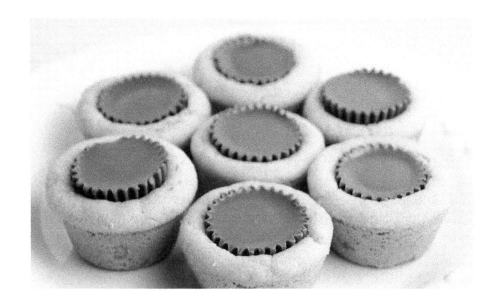

Curry ` n Poppy Devilled Eggs

Prep Time:
20 Minutes
Cook Time:
8 Minutes
Serve: 6

Ingredients:

- ½ cup mayonnaise
- ½ tbsp poppy seeds
- 1 tbsp red curry paste
- 6 eggs
- ¼ tsp salt

Directions:

1.Place eggs in a small pot and add enough water to cover it. Bring to a boil without a cover, lower fire to a simmer and simmer for 8 minutes.

2.Immediately dunk in ice cold water once done cooking. Peel eggshells and slice eggs in half lengthwise.

3.Remove yolks and place them in a medium bowl. Add the rest of the ingredients in the bowl except for the egg whites. Mix well.

4.Evenly return the yolk mixture into the middle of the egg whites.

Nutrition: Calories: 200; Fat: 19.0g; Carbs: 1.0g; Protein: 6.0g

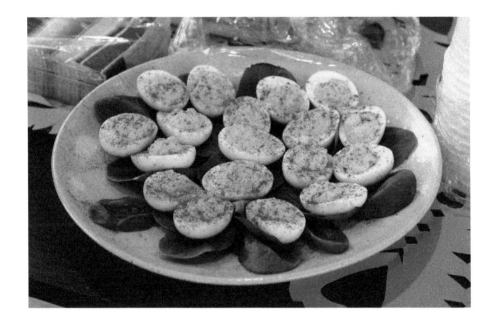

Potato Mash

Prep Time:

15 minutes

Cook Time:

20 minutes

Serve: 32

Ingredients:

- 10 large baking potatoes, peeled and cubed
- 3 tablespoons organic olive oil, divided
- 1 onion, chopped
- 1 tablespoon ground turmeric
- ½ teaspoon ground cumin
- Salt and freshly ground black pepper, to taste

Directions:

1.In a large pan of water, add potatoes and produce with a boil on medium-high heat.

2.Cook approximately twenty or so minutes.

3.Drain well and transfer in to a large bowl.

4.With a potato masher, mash the potatoes.

5.Meanwhile in a very skillet, heat 1 tablespoon of oil on medium-high heat.

6.Add onion and sauté for about 6 minutes.

7.Add onion mixture in the bowl with mashed potatoes.

8.Add turmeric, cumin, salt and black pepper and mash till well combined.
9.Stir in remaining oil and serve.

Nutrition: Calories: 103, Fat: 1.4g, Carbohydrates: 21.3g, Fiber: 2g, Protein: 1.8g

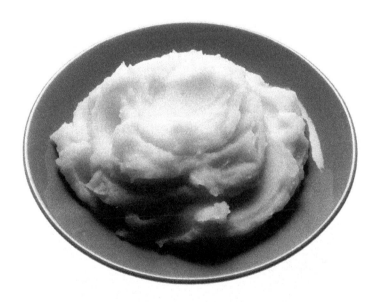

Creamy Sweet Potato Mash

Prep Time:
15 minutes
Cook Time:
21 minutes
Serve: 4

Ingredients:

- 1 tbsp. extra virgin olive oil
- 2 large sweet potatoes, peeled and chopped
- 2 teaspoons ground turmeric
- 1 garlic herb, minced
- 2 cups vegetable broth
- 2 tablespoons unsweetened coconut milk Salt and freshly ground black pepper, to taste Chopped pistachios, for garnishing

Directions:

1.In a big skillet, heat oil on medium-high heat.
Add sweet potato and stir fry for bout 2-3 minutes.

2.Add turmeric and stir fry for approximately 1 minute.

3.Add garlic and stir fry approximately 2 minutes.

4.Add broth and provide to a boil.

5.Reduce the heat to low and cook for approximately 10-15 minutes or till

6.every one of the liquids is absorbed.

7.Transfer the sweet potato mixture in to a bowl.

8.Add coconut milk, salt and black pepper and mash it completely.
9.Garnish with pistachio and serve.

Nutrition: Calories: 110, Fat: 5g, Carbohydrates: 16g, Protein: 1g

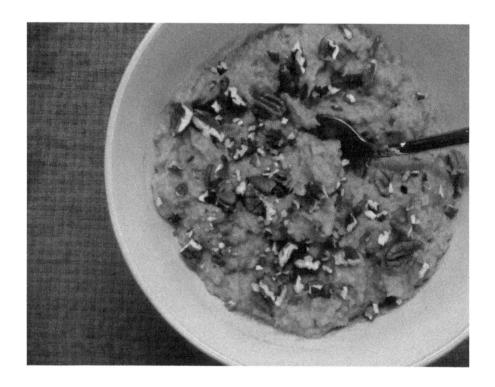

Gingered Cauliflower Rice

Prep Time:
15 minutes
Cook Time:
10 min
Serve: 3-4

Ingredients:

- 3 tablespoons coconut oil
- 4 (1/8-inch thickfresh ginger slices
- 1 small head cauliflower, trimmed and processed into rice consistency
- 3 garlic cloves, crushed
- 1 tablespoon chives, chopped
- 1 tablespoon coconut vinegar
- Salt, to taste

Directions:

1.In a skillet, melt coconut oil on medium-high heat.

2.Add ginger and sauté for about 2-3 minutes.

3.Discard the ginger slices and stir in cauliflower and garlic.

4.Cook, stirring occasionally approximately 7-8 minutes.

5.Stir in remaining ingredients and take off from heat.

Nutrition: Calories: 67, Fat: 3.5g, Carbohydrates: 4.5g, Fiber: 2g, Protein: 7g

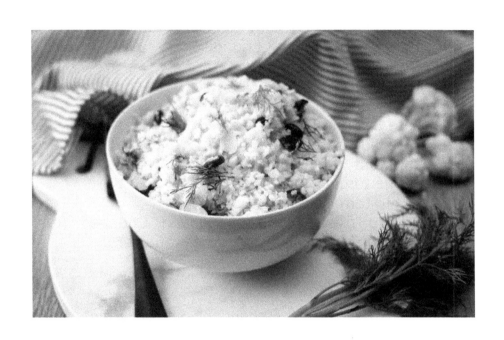

Spicy Cauliflower Rice

Prep Time:
15 minutes
Cook Time:
10 minutes
Serve: 4

Ingredients:

- 3 tablespoons coconut oil
- 1 small white onion, chopped
- 3 garlic cloves, minced
- 1 large head cauliflower, trimmed and processed into rice consistency
- ½ teaspoon ground cumin
- ½ teaspoon paprika
- Salt and freshly ground black pepper, to taste 1large tomato, chopped
- ¼ cup tomato paste
- ¼ cup fresh cilantro, chopped Chopped fresh cilantro, for garnishing 2 limes, quarters

Directions:

1.In a sizable skillet, melt coconut oil on medium-high heat.

2.Add onion and sauté for approximately 2 minutes.

3.Add garlic and sauté approximately 1 minute.

4.Stir in cauliflower rice.

5.Add cumin, paprika, salt and black pepper and cook, stirring occasionally approximately 2-3 minutes.

6.Stir in tomato, tomato paste and cilantro and cook approximately 2-3 minutes.

7.Garnish with cilantro and serve alongside lime.

Nutrition: Calories: 246, Fat: 11g, Carbohydrates: 26g, Fiber: 4g, Protein: 21g

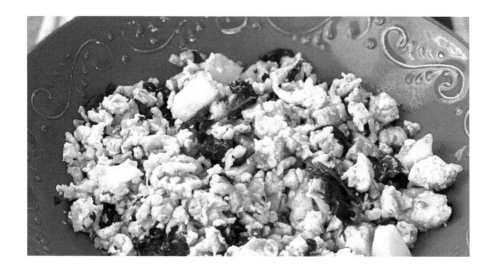

Simple Brown Rice

Prep Time:
10 minutes
Cook Time:
50 minutes
Serve: 4

Ingredients:

- 1 cup brown rice
- 2 cups chicken broth
- 1 tablespoon ground turmeric
- 1 tbsp. extra virgin olive oil

Directions:

1.In a pan, add rice, broth and turmeric and provide with a boil.

2.Reduce the warmth to low.

3.Simmer, covered for about 50 minutes.

4.Add the organic olive oil and fluff using a fork.

5.Keep aside, covered approximately 10 minutes before.

Nutrition: Calories: 320, Fat: 6g, Carbohydrates: 285g, Fiber: 4g, Protein: 21g

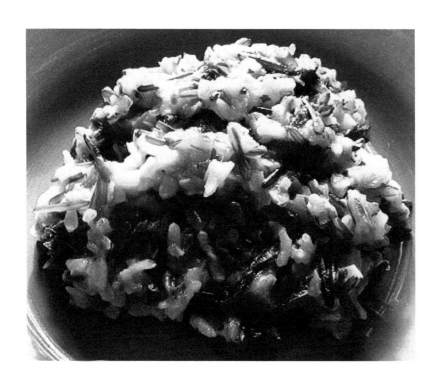

Spicy Quinoa

Prep Time:
10 minutes
Cook Time:
25 minutes
Serve: 4

Ingredients:

- 2 tablespoons extra-virgin essential olive oil
- 1 teaspoon curry powder
- 1 teaspoon ground turmeric
- 12 teaspoon ground cumin
- 1 cup quinoa, rinsed and drained
- 2 cups chicken broth
- ¾ cup almonds, toasted
- ½ cup raisins
- ¾ cup fresh parsley, chopped

Directions:

1. In a medium pan, heat oil on medium-low heat.

2. Add curry powder, turmeric and cumin and sauté for approximately 1-2 minutes.

3. Add quinoa and sauté approximately 2-3 minutes.

4. Add broth and stir to blend.

5. Cover reducing the warmth to low.

6. Simmer for around twenty minutes.

7.Remove from heat while aside, covered approximately 5 minutes.

8.Just before, add almonds and raisins and toss to coat.
9.10Drizzle with lemon juice and serve.

Nutrition: Calories: 237, Fat: 3g, Carbohydrates: 17g, Fiber: 6g, Protein: 31g

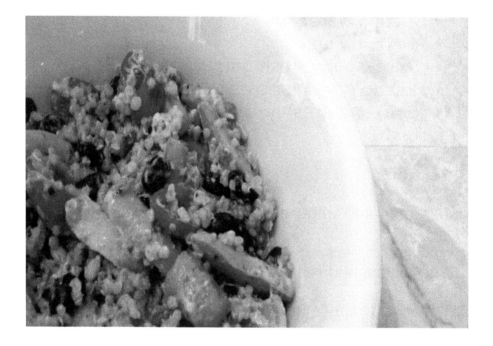

Quinoa with Apricots

Prep Time:
15 minutes
Cook Time:
12 minutes
Serve: 4

Ingredients:

- 2 cups water
- 1 cup quinoa
- ½ teaspoon fresh ginger, grated finely
- ½ cup dried apricots, chopped roughly
- Salt and freshly ground black pepper, to taste

Directions:

1.In a pan, add water on high heat and bring to your boil.

2.Add quinoa and reduce the heat to medium.

3.Cover and reduce the heat to low.

4.Simmer for about 12 minutes.

5.Remove from heat and immediately, stir in ginger and apricots. Keep aside, covered for approximately fifteen minutes before.

Nutrition: Calories: 267, Fat: 3.5g, Carbohydrates: 4g, Fiber: 5g, Protein: 17g

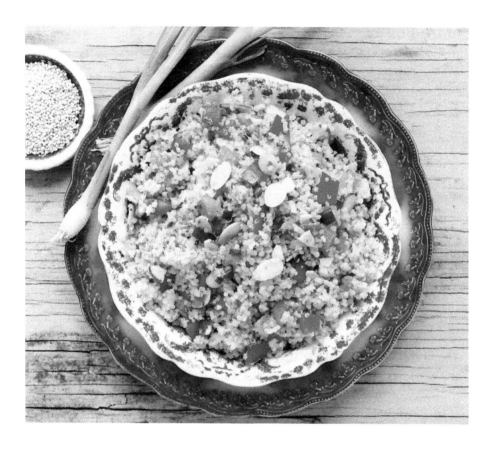

Easy Zucchini Slaw

Prep Time:
10 minutes
Serve: 3

Ingredients:

- 2 tablespoons extra-virgin olive oil
- 1 zucchini, shredded
- 1 teaspoon Dijon mustard
- 1 yellow bell pepper, sliced
- 1 red onion, thinly sliced

Directions:

1.Combine all ingredients in a salad bowl. Season with the salt and black pepper to taste.

2.Let it sit in your refrigerator for about 1 hour before.

Nutrition: 96 Calories; 9.4g Fat; 2.8g Carbs; 0.7g Protein; 0.4g Fiber Ingredients

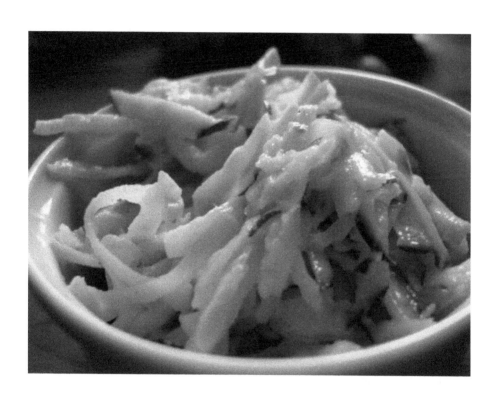

Broc n' Cheese

Prep Time:
25 minutes
Serve: 5

Ingredients:

- 1 ½ pounds broccoli florets
- 3 tablespoons olive oil
- 1/2 cup cream of mushrooms soup
- 1 teaspoon garlic, minced
- 6 ounces Swiss cheese, shredded

Directions:

1.Start by preheating your oven to 380 degrees F. Brush the sides and bottom of a baking dish with 1 tablespoon olive oil.

2.In a small nonstick skillet, heat 1 tablespoon of the olive oil over a moderate heat. Sauté the garlic for 30 seconds or until just beginning to brown.

3.In a soup pot, parboil the broccoli until crisp-tender; place the rinsed broccoli in the prepared baking dish. Place the sautéed garlic on top. Drizzle the remaining tablespoon of olive oil over everything.

4.Season with the salt and black pepper. Pour in the cream of mushroom soup.

5.2Top with the Swiss cheese.

6.Bake for 20 minutes until the cheese is hot and bubbly.

Nutrition: 179 Calories; 10.3g Fat; 7.6g Carbs; 13.5g
Protein; 3.6g Fiber

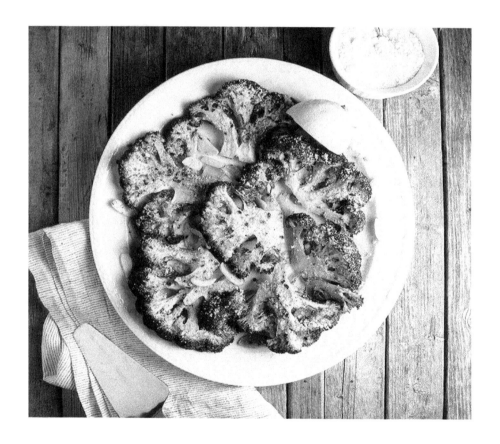

Greek Avgolemono Soup

Prep Time:
25 minutes
Serve: 6

Ingredients:

- 1 pound fennel bulbs, sliced
- 1 celery stalk, chopped
- 1 tablespoon freshly squeezed lemon juice
- 2 eggs
- 5 cups chicken stock

Directions:

1.Heat 2 tablespoons of olive oil in a soup pot over medium-high heat. Sauté the fennel and celery until tender but not browned, approximately 7 minutes.

2.Add in Mediterranean seasoning mix and continue to sauté until they are fragrant.

3.Add in the chicken stock and bring to a rapid boil. Turn the temperature to medium-low; let it simmer for 10 to 13 minutes.

4.Puree your soup using a food processor or an immersion blender.

5.Thoroughly whisk the eggs and lemon juice until well combined; pour 2 cups of the hot soup into the egg mixture, whisking continuously.

6.Return the mixture to the pot; continue cooking for 2 to 3 minutes more until cooked through. Spoon into individual bowls.

Nutrition: 86 Calories; 6.1g Fat; 6g Carbs; 2.8g Protein; 2.4g Fiber

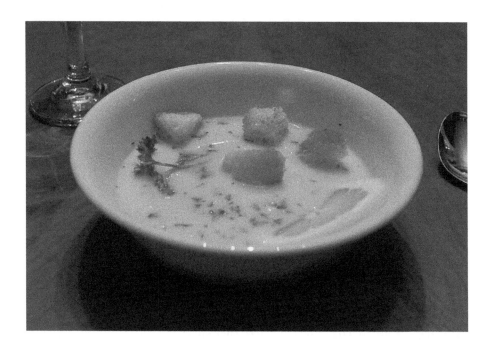

Italian Zuppa Di Pomodoro

Prep Time:
35 minutes
Serve: 4

Ingredients:

- 1/2 cup scallions, chopped
- 1 ½ pounds Roma tomatoes, diced
- 2 cups Brodo di Pollo (Italian broth
- 2 tablespoons tomato paste
- 2 cups mustard greens, torn into pieces

Directions:

1.Heat 2 teaspoon of olive oil in a large pot over medium-high heat. Sauté the scallions for 2 to 3 minutes until tender.

2.Add in Roma tomatoes, Italian broth, and tomato paste
and bring to a boil. Reduce the temperature to medium-low and continue to simmer, partially covered, for about 25 minutes.

3.Puree the soup with an immersion blender and return it to the pot. Add in the mustard greens and continue to cook until the greens wilt.

4.Taste, adjust seasonings and serve immediately.

Nutrition: 104 Calories; 7.2g Fat; 6.2g Carbs; 2.6g Protein; 3.1g Fiber

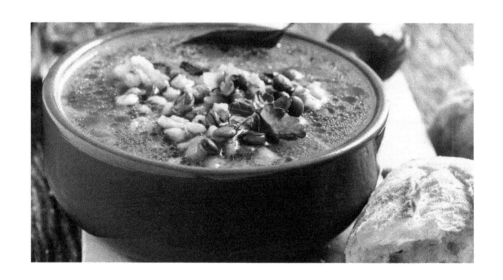

Easy Zucchini Croquets

Prep Time:
40 minutes
Serve: 6

Ingredients:

- 1 egg
- 1/2 cup almond meal
- 1 pound zucchini, grated and drained
- 1/2 cup goat cheese, crumbled
- 2 tablespoons olive oil

Directions:

1.Combine the egg, almond milk, zucchini and cheese in a mixing bowl.

2.Refrigerate the mixture for 20 to 30 minutes.

3.Heat the oil in a frying pan over medium-high heat. Scoop the heaped tablespoons of the mixture into the hot oil.

4.Cook for about 4 minutes per side; cook in batches.

Nutrition: 111 Calories; 8.9g Fat; 3.2g Carbs; 5.8g Protein; 1g Fiber

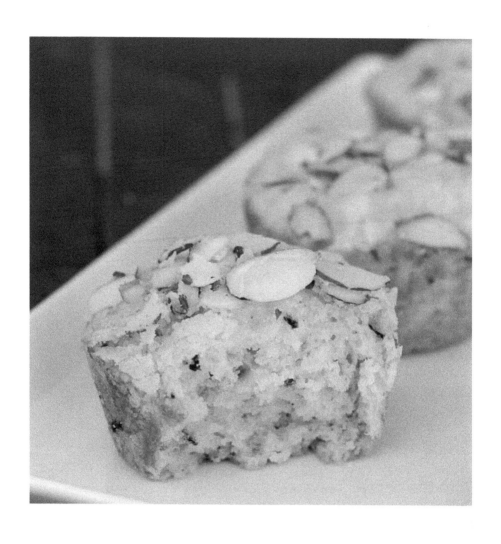

Pork and Cheese Stuffed Peppers

Prep Time:
30 minutes
Serve: 2

Ingredients:

- 2 sweet Italian peppers, deveined and halved
- 1/2 Spanish onion, finely chopped
- 1 cup marinara sauce
- 1/2 cup cheddar cheese, grated
- 4 ounces pork, ground

Directions:

1.Heat 1 tablespoon of canola oil in a saucepan over a moderate heat. Then, sauté the onion for 3 to 4 minutes until tender and fragrant.

2.Add in the ground pork; cook for 3 to 4 minutes more. Add in Italian seasoning mix. Spoon the mixture into the pepper halves.

3.Spoon the marinara sauce into a lightly greased baking dish. Arrange the stuffed peppers in the baking dish.

4.Bake in the preheated oven at 395 degrees F for 17 to 20 minutes. Top with cheddar cheese and continue to bake for about 5 minutes or until the top is golden brown. Bon appétit!

Nutrition: 313 Calories; 21.3g Fat; 5.7g Carbs; 20.2g Protein; 1.9g Fiber

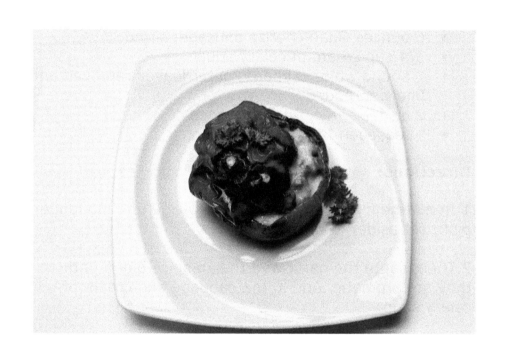

Stewed Cabbage with Goan Chorizo Sausage

Prep Time:
30 minutes
Serve: 3

Ingredients:

- 6 ounces Goan chorizo sausage, sliced
- 3/4 cup cream of celery soup
- 1 pound white cabbage, outer leaves removed and finely shredded
- 2 cloves garlic, finely chopped
- 1 teaspoon Indian spice blend

Directions:

1.In a large frying pan, sear the sausage until no longer pink; set aside.

2.Then, sauté the garlic and Indian spice blend until they are aromatic. Add in the cabbage and cream of celery soup.

3.Turn the heat to simmer; continue to simmer, partially covered, for about 20 minutes or until cooked through.

4.Top with the reserved Goan chorizo sausage and serve.

Nutrition: 235 Calories; 17.7g Fat; 6.1g Carbs; 9.8g Protein; 2.4g Fiber

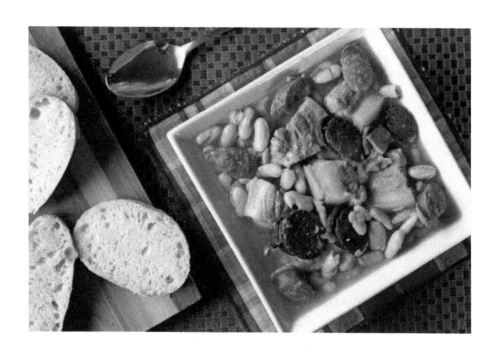

Cauliflower and Ham Casserole

Prep Time:
10 minutes
Serve: 6

Ingredients:

- 1 ½ pounds cauliflower, broken into small florets
- 6 ounces ham, diced
- 4 eggs, beaten
- 1/2 cup Greek-Style yogurt
- 1 cup Swiss cheese, preferably freshly grated

Directions:

1.Parboil the cauliflower in a saucepan for about 10 minutes or until tender.

2.Drain and puree in your food processor.

3.Add in the ham, eggs, and Greek-Style yogurt; stir to combine well.

4.Spoon the mixture into a lightly buttered baking dish. Top with the Swiss cheese and bake in the preheated oven at 385 degrees F for about 20 minutes.

Nutrition: 236 Calories; 13.8g Fat; 7.2g Carbs; 20.3g Protein; 2.3g Fiber

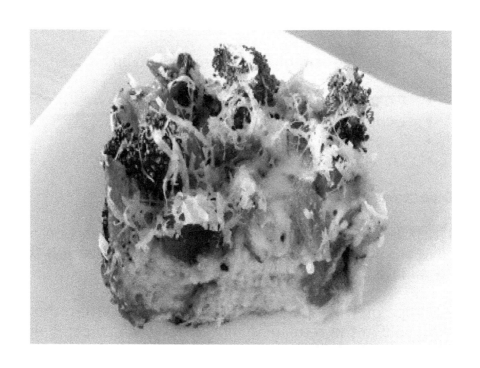

Stuffed Spaghetti Squash

Prep Time:
1 hour
Serve: 4

Ingredients:

- ½ pound spaghetti squash, halved, scoop out seeds
- 1 garlic clove, minced
- 1 cup cream cheese
- 2 eggs
- 1/2 cup Mozzarella cheese, shredded

Directions:

1.Drizzle the insides of each squash with 1 teaspoon of olive oil. Bake in the preheated oven at 380 degrees for 45 minutes.

2.Scrape out the spaghetti squash "noodles" from the skin. Fold in the remaining ingredients; stir to combine well.

3.Spoon the cheese mixture into squash halves. Bake at 360 degrees for about 9 minutes, until the cheese is hot and bubbly.

Nutrition: 219 Calories; 17.5g Fat; 6.9g Carbs; 9g Protein; 0.9g Fiber

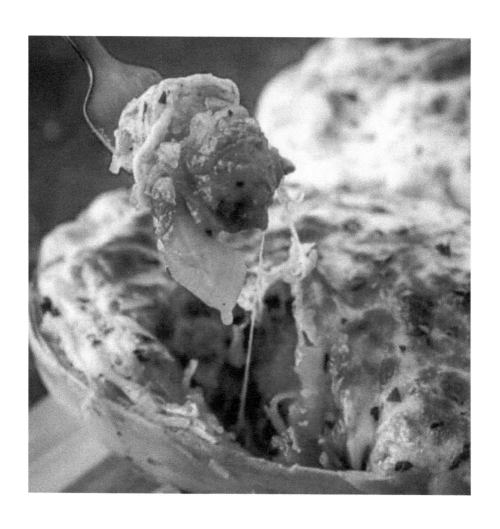

Spicy and Warm Coleslaw

Prep Time:
45 minutes
Serve: 4

Ingredients:

- 1 medium-sized leek, chopped
- 1 tablespoon balsamic vinegar
- 1 teaspoon yellow mustard
- ½ pound green cabbage, shredded
- ½ teaspoon Sriracha sauce

Directions:

1.Drizzle 2 tablespoons of the olive oil over the leek and cabbage; sprinkle with salt and black pepper.

2.Bake in the preheated oven at 410 degrees F for about 40 minutes. Transfer the mixture to a salad bowl.

3.Toss with 1 tablespoon of olive oil, mustard, balsamic vinegar, and Sriracha sauce. Serve warm!

Nutrition: 118 Calories; 10.2g Fat; 6.6g Carbs; 1.1g Protein; 1.9g Fiber

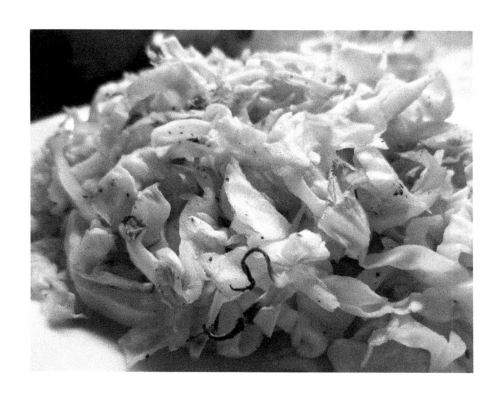

Easy Mediterranean Croquettes

Prep Time:
40minutes
Serve: 2

Ingredients:

- ½ pound zucchini, grated
- ½ cup Swiss cheese, shredded
- 3 eggs, whisked Mediterranean
- 1/3 cup almond meal
- 2 tablespoons pork rinds

Directions:

1.Place the grated zucchini in a colander, sprinkle with 1/2 teaspoon of salt, and let it stand for 30 minutes. Drain the zucchini well and discard any excess water.

2.Heat 2 tablespoons of olive oil in a frying pan over medium-high heat. Mix the zucchini with the remaining ingredients until well combined.

3.Shape the mixture into croquettes and cook for 2 to 3 minutes per side. Enjoy!

Nutrition: 463 Calories; 36g Fat; 7.6g Carbs; 27.5g Protein; 2.8g Fiber

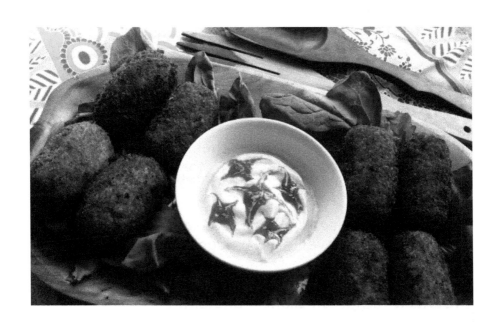

Tuscan Asparagus with Cheese

Prep Time:
20 minutes
Serve: 5

Ingredients:

- 1 ½ pounds asparagus, trimmed
- 1 tablespoon Sriracha sauce
- 1 tablespoon fresh cilantro, roughly chopped
- 4 tablespoons Pecorino Romano cheese, grated
- 4 tablespoons butter, melted

Directions:

1.Toss the asparagus with the cheese, melted butter, and Sriracha sauce; season with Italian spice mix, if desired.

2.Arrange your asparagus on a baking sheet and roast in the preheated oven at 410 degrees for 12 to 15 minutes.

3.Garnish with fresh cilantro and enjoy!

Nutrition: 140 Calories; 11.5g Fat; 5.5g Carbs; 5.6g Protein; 2.9g Fiber

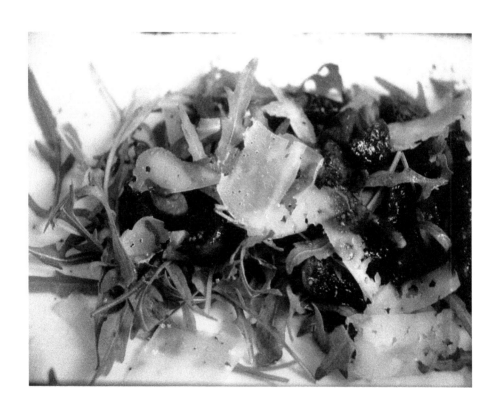

Brown Mushroom Stew

Prep Time:
20 minutes
Serve: 6

Ingredients:

- 2 pounds brown mushrooms, sliced
- 1 bell pepper, sliced
- 2 cups chicken broth
- ½ cup leeks, finely diced
- 1 cup herb-infused tomato sauce

Directions:

1.Heat 4 tablespoons of oil in a soup pot over a moderate flame. Sauté the pepper and leeks for about 4 to 5 minutes.

2.Stir in the mushrooms and continue to sauté for about 2 minutes. Pour in a splash of broth to deglaze the bottom of the pan.

3.After that, add in the tomato sauce and the remaining broth; bring to a boil.

4.Turn the heat to simmer.

5.Continue to cook, partially covered, for about 10 minutes or until the mushrooms are tender and thoroughly cooked.

6.Ladle into soup bowls and serve. Bon appétit!

Nutrition: 123 Calories; 9.2g Fat; 5.8g Carbs; 4.7g Protein; 1.4g Fiber

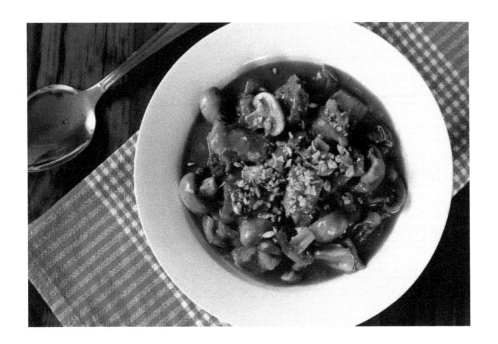

Wax Beans in Wine Sauce

Prep Time:
15 minutes
Serve: 4

Ingredients:

- ½ pound wax beans, trimmed
- 2 tablespoons dry white wine
- 1 tablespoon butter
- ½ teaspoon mustard seeds
- ½ cup tomato sauce with garlic and onions

Directions:

1.Melt the butter in a soup pot over medium-high heat. Then, fry wax beans in hot butter for 2 to 3 minutes.

2.Add in tomato sauce, wine, and mustard seeds; season with salt and black pepper.

3.Turn the temperature to medium-low and continue to simmer for about 8 longer or until wax beans are tender and the sauce has thickened slightly. Bon appétit!

Nutrition: 56 Calories; 3.5g Fat; 6g Carbs; 1.5g Protein; 2.2g Fiber

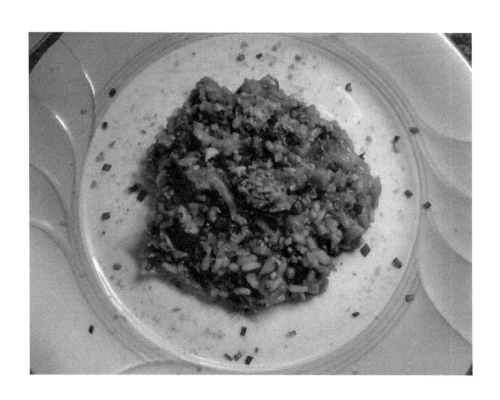

Lebanese Mushroom Stew with Za'atar

Prep Time:
1 hour 50 minutes
Serve: 4

Ingredients:

- 8 ounces Chanterelle mushroom, sliced
- 1 cup tomato sauce with onion and garlic
- 4 tablespoons olive oil
- 2 bell peppers, chopped
- ½ teaspoon Za'atar spice

Directions:

1.Heat olive oil in a heavy-bottomed pot over medium-high heat. Once hot, sauté the peppers until tender or about 3 minutes.

2.Stir in the mushrooms and continue to sauté until they have softened

3.Add in Za'atar spice and tomato sauce; bring to a rapid boil. Immediately, turn the heat to medium-low.

4.Continue to simmer for about 35 minutes until cooked through. Bon appétit!

Nutrition: 155 Calories; 13.9g Fat; 6g Carbs; 1.4g Protein; 2.9g Fiber

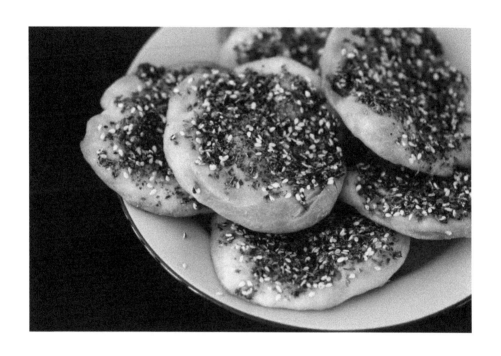

Skinny Cucumber Noodles with Sauce

Prep Time:
35 minutes
Serve: 2

Ingredients:

- 1 cucumber, spiralized
- ½ teaspoon sea salt
- 1 tablespoon olive oil
- 1 tablespoon fresh lime juice
- 1 California avocado, pitted, peeled and mashed

Directions:

1.Sprinkle your cucumber with salt; let it stand for 30 minutes; after that, discard the excess water and pat the cucumber dry with kitchen towels.

2.In the meantime, combine olive oil, lime juice, and avocado. Season with salt and black pepper.

3.Toss the cucumber noodles with sauce and serve. Bon appétit!

Nutrition: 194 Calories; 17.1g Fat; 7.6g Carbs; 2.5g Protein; 4.6g Fiber

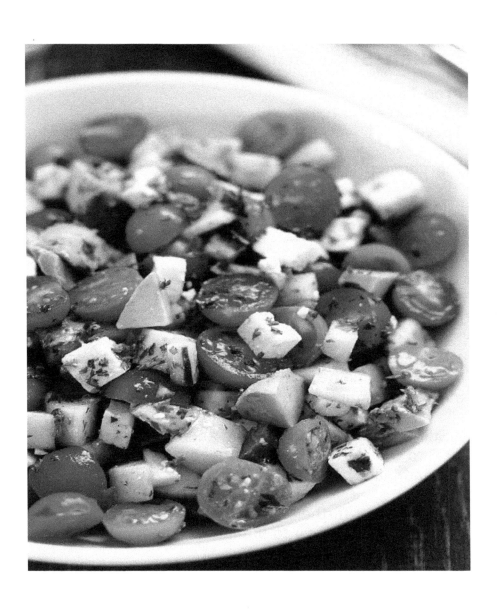

Balkan-Style Stir-Fry

Prep Time:
25 minutes
Serve: 5

Ingredients:

- 8 bell peppers, deveined and cut into strips
- 1 tomato, chopped
- 2 eggs
- 1 yellow onion, sliced
- 3 garlic cloves, halved

Directions:

1.Heat 2 tablespoons of olive oil in a saucepan over medium-low flame. Sweat the onion for about 4 minutes or until tender and translucent.

2.Stir in the garlic and peppers and continue to sauté for 5 to 6 minutes. Fold in chopped tomato along with salt and black pepper.

3.Stir fry for a further 7 minutes. Stir in the eggs and continue to cook for 4 to 5 minutes longer. Serve immediately.

Nutrition: 114 Calories; 7.6g Fat; 6g Carbs; 3.4g Protein; 1.5g Fiber

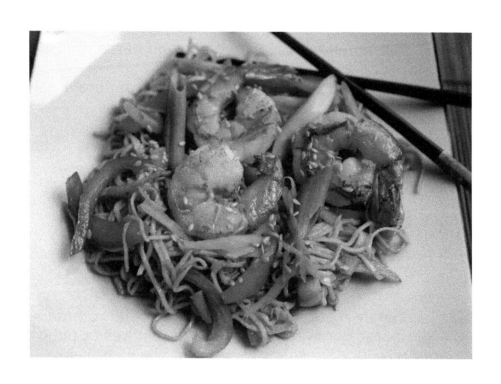

Italian Zoodles with Romano Cheese

Prep Time:
15 minutes
Serve: 3

Ingredients:

- 1 ½ tablespoons olive oil
- 3 cups button mushrooms, chopped
- 1 cup tomato sauce with garlic and herbs
- 1 pound zucchini, spiralized
- 1/3 cup Pecorino Romano cheese, preferably freshly grated

Directions:

1.In a saucepan, heat the olive oil over a moderate heat. Once hot, cook the mushrooms for about 4 minutes until they have softened.

2.Stir in the tomato sauce and zucchini, bringing to a boil.

3.Immediately reduce temperature to simmer. Continue to cook, partially covered, for about 7 minutes or until cooked through. Season with salt and black pepper.

4.Top with Pecorino Romano cheese and serve. Bon appétit!

Nutrition: 160 Calories; 10.6g Fat; 7.4g Carbs; 10g Protein; 3.4g Fiber

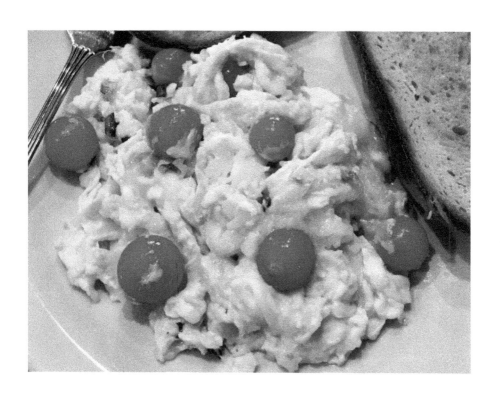

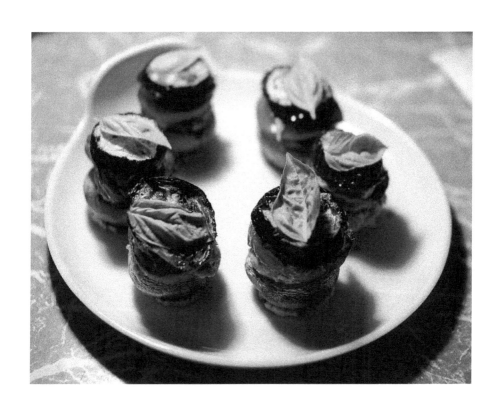

Lightning Source UK Ltd.
Milton Keynes UK
UKHW051638090621
385195UK00006B/22